ULTIMATE Intimacy

ULTIMATE
Intimacy

The
Revolutionary
Science of
Female
Sexual Health

CAROLYN A. DELUCIA
MD, FACOG

NEW YORK

LONDON • NASHVILLE • MELBOURNE • VANCOUVER

Ultimate Intimacy

The Revolutionary Science of Female Sexual Health

© 2021 Carolyn DeLucia, MD FACOG

All rights reserved. No portion of this book may be reproduced, stored in a retrieval system, or transmitted in any form or by any means—electronic, mechanical, photocopy, recording, scanning, or other—except for brief quotations in critical reviews or articles, without the prior written permission of the publisher.

Published in New York, New York, by Morgan James Publishing in partnership with Difference Press. Morgan James is a trademark of Morgan James, LLC. www.MorganJamesPublishing.com

ISBN 9781642799217 paperback
ISBN 9781642799224 eBook
ISBN 9781642799231 audiobook
Library of Congress Control Number: 2019956203

Cover Design Concept:
Jennifer Stimson

Editor:
Moriah Howell

Cover & Interior Design by:
Christopher Kirk
www.GFSstudio.com

Coaching:
Author Incubator

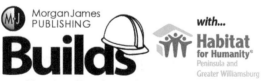

Morgan James is a proud partner of Habitat for Humanity Peninsula and Greater Williamsburg. Partners in building since 2006.
Get involved today! Visit
MorganJamesPublishing.com/giving-back

DISCLAIMER The knowledge that is derived from this book is in no way to replace personal medical advice from your doctor. It is merely information about techniques that the author has discovered through treatment of her own patients. She has learned that each patient is an individual, and therefore each person must get attention for their particular condition. Neither the author nor the publisher takes any responsibility for omissions, errors, or misinterpretation of the medical information in this book. Any such situation is unintentional

I dedicate this book to my amazing daughters,
who are incredible women leaving my true
footprint on this earth.
May they always be empowered and fulfilled.

Table of Contents

PART 1

Chapter 1
My Sex Life Is Over

It has been weeks now. With each passing day and with each rejection, you are getting more and more anxious. You lay awake fretting that your partner, Nick, will cheat, or leave you. You cannot bear the pain of having sex. You are so scared, and you do not know what to do, so you make an emergency appointment with the GYN.

The doctor explains that after menopause, you can feel dry. At first, you feel so relieved that it is not that something had changed subconsciously about how you feel about Nick. The doctor says you can try lubricants or some local hormone therapy. He explains that the cream form could be sloppy but may help. You are hesitant to use hormones because your mother had breast cancer at fifty-five years old. That is not an option in your mind.

But you still hope the lubricant would help. Maybe you are just frightened, and it was not as bad as you remember. You are anxious to try the lubricant, but since it has never been an issue, you struggle with how to bring it up to Nick. How can you be so nervous to talk about this with the partner you have been with for decades?! You feel isolated and alone. You torment over what to say to Nick. Why had you not known this could happen? Why had no one ever discussed this? Why do women share horror stories about childbirth but not share what happens when you get older? Why? Because it is too horrible to utter. It has terrible consequences on your life. It is tearing your marriage apart.

What if the lubricant doesn't help? What if you can't have sex ever again? Will you have to give oral pleasures for the rest of your married life? You don't hate it, but what's in it for you? On top of that, reaching climax is taking forever. At some point during sex, you begin thinking of what you'll make for dinner the next evening and have to pull yourself back to the moment. There is so little sensation that Nick could have been rubbing your forehead instead. In horror, it pains you to think of the most embarrassing issue of all! You feel sometimes like you cannot hold your urine and may leak not only when you run, but during sex! How humiliating! What kind of turn off that is? You are almost too afraid to relax and enjoy the moment for fear of losing control.

Is he revolted by this? Do you not find him attractive anymore? Are you going to feel unconnected to Nick? Will he get mad at you? Is he already looking elsewhere? He has been mentioning how helpful his assistant is. He spends more time with her each day than he does with you. The sickening feeling in the pit of your stomach is too much to bear. Would he meet a new, younger woman and leave you? Oh my gosh, are you going to lose your husband? You have always been so sexual, and you know how important this is to him. It is important to you, too. Being intimate has always made you feel so close to Nick. Making love is his favorite way to show his love for you. Without that, what will happen? You're desperate for answers. You stay awake at night crying, especially after rejecting his advances once again and hearing him sigh in disappointment.

That's when it hits you. Why have you not thought to google this? But, google what? "Losing your husband over fifty?" "Is lack of sex why the divorce rate is so high?" "How to give an amazing blow job?" "Never orgasming?" "Where to buy lubricant goo?" "Broken vagina?"

You could just call your bestie and see if she has a broken vagina, too. But how do you bring up the topic? The last time you ever mentioned sex, you had debated if fantasizing during sex was cheating. You never really get that personal. Feeling frustrated and convinced you are the only one in this position with no one to share these feelings with and will soon surely lose your husband, you open the computer.

You google divorce first.... infidelity is the number one cause of divorce today! You switch gears and look up lubricants. But there are so many, you may need a PhD to figure out which is best. Oops! Now you are on a porn site!

What will Nick think if he looks up your history? Now you are blushing, and your palms are sweating. Hit the back arrow! Okay, back to original search. You laugh; looks like they have WD-40 and Anti-Seize on the same page as personal lubricants. You need the giggle. You go for it and google "broken vagina." Well look at this! You are not alone, but some of these options are scary! Physical therapy, hormones, loose vaginas, women leaking urine. This could be much worse than you even imagined. You slam the computer closed. What does all this mean? What pertains to you? Who can you talk to? Lost, alone, confused, frightened, and desperate! Your vagina is broken!

You try one more time, google "painful sex," and a new category pops up. "Female sexual health" seems to be a new growing topic. You just have never really heard of any of these procedures or treatments. They sound promising and encouraging; certainly, better than the solutions the doctor has offered so far. From testimonials, you see that women have had great success. They are having painless and enjoyable sex. They are sharing the changes in their lives from having a healthy sex life with their partners. Whether in a homosexual or heterosexual relationship, intimacy is the glue that holds it together. With the security of a fulfilling home life, things are changing in the rest of their lives. The ripple effect is amazing! The kids are more stable and feel the contentment in the family, spurring them on to excel. At work, they feel less stressed and more confident. Yes! They feel empowered. Taking control of your personal health, improving your interpersonal relationships with conviction, affects every aspect of your life! It just may be your time to look into some new ways to address these issues before it is too late.

Chapter 2

Journey Into the Vagina Revolution

Allow me to introduce myself…

I am a woman of education, of great taste, of experience, and I desire to change your life. I am fifty-six years young and have been practicing medicine for over thirty years. I chose obstetrics and gynecology because I find the field rewarding. No matter what ails a woman, a gynecologist can either treat it with hormones or perform a procedure to fix it. There seemed to be a solution, if not a cure, for anything that sickens the female body.

Over the years, I personally experienced a lot of the changes that women inevitably have through life. I got married right out of medical school to a fellow student. We jumped into our careers and were newlyweds all in the same week. Our first year was tumultuous, and by the third year of marriage, with both working over 70 hours a week and I was pregnant with our first child. To no one's surprise, I went into preterm labor. My beautiful baby was born at thirty-six weeks, but was healthy and strong. Three years later, after two miscarriages, I had my second daughter. We raised our daughters over the next several years, both working terrible hours. When my eldest was ten, she had a piano recital that I was aware of, but with a patient in labor and one hour to spare I hoped to be able to accomplish both. I gambled that I could deliver the baby and get to the recital in time. My daughter, in all her wisdom said, "Mommy, if you are not in the audience, I am not going on that stage." I arrived five minutes after her time slot to find out she did not perform.

That was a pivotal moment. I did not have children to have a nanny raise them, and I did not want to miss out on the special moments in their lives. Something had to change! I discussed stopping the obstetrical portion of my practice with my husband and we decided that I would stop doing deliveries and focus on gynecology. My income dropped in half, as would be expected, putting a strain on the marriage as financial stress often does. So, we explored secondary ways of creating an income.

This is how I discovered the world of cosmetic medicine. I started in 2002 with laser hair reduction and cosmetic Botox. I enjoyed the creativity of aesthetic medicine, and by 2014 had a full- service medical spa in NJ, ViVa Rejuvenation Center. Then one day, a handsome device salesman walked in, representing a company that had modified its facial laser for use in the vagina! At first, I was skeptical but when he mentioned the possible improvement in urinary incontinence and vaginal dryness, my interest piqued. I purchased the laser and, true to their word, my patients were experiencing improvement in their symptoms of urinary leakage and vaginal atrophy. I was changing lives. And since it was the first laser of its kind in the North East, I had patients traveling from all over to get treatments.

My next step was to explore what else was on the horizon in the field of female sexual health. I traveled to Fairhope, Alabama to meet and learn from the genius Charles Runels, MD. He is the inventor of the O-Shot™ as well as all the Vampire procedures™. The ability to enhance sensation with this simple procedure worked very well in combination with the laser treatments. It was at this point that I realized what an impact this could have on women. Being menopausal myself and having experienced excruciating pain with sex and loss of sensation making it near impossible to climax, I volunteered to be the first guinea pig. Since it worked for me then, it could work for other women, too. More doctors need to know how to do these procedures, and more women need to be aware they exist. I became faculty with the Cellular Medicine Association and the American Aesthetic Association and started teaching physicians worldwide.

Around the same time, Cindy Barshop of Real Housewives of New York had been following the evolution of the vaginal lasers. She had created an empire with her string of spas in New York City know as Completely Bare, which had focused on hair reduction. She decided to try her brilliance in the field of female sexual health, so she visited me in New Jersey to discuss the possibility of creating a safe haven for women using the new tools I had discovered. She founded VSPOT Medispa, and I quickly joined her. We have successfully established a location

Chapter 3
Vagina is the New Kale

– Emily Morse

The vagina has been prodded, poked, stretched, and even revered. Now after all the abuse, it no longer feels the same during intimacy. There is either loss of sensation or lack of arousal and pleasure. There is pain and friction that feels like sandpaper scratching the inside walls. Without knowledge of how to correct this, it may get worse over time. It might even have a divisive effect on your relationship. This book helps to explore the options available to address each of these issues. The non-medical therapies, as well as the surgical and non-invasive procedures will be explored, giving you the tools you need to make the best choice for you at this time in order to maintain your sexual health.

The suffering is very real, but finally, there are answers. There are ways to feel better and solve the problems holding you back from engaging in the intimacy you so desire.

Imagine being able to relax and accept the advances of your partner. Imagine not feeling pain, but instead feeling pleasure better than you thought possible. The result of healthy intimate relationships has a ripple effect on the rest of your life. The calming effect of sexual pleasure improves rest. Being alert and ready to take on the world in the morning makes you able to do any task that comes your way that much more efficiently. Doing your job better may lead to further success and satisfaction in your career. Furthermore, children always know when their parents are happy together and present as a united front. This is healthy for children, and they flourish in a secure environment. All of this may seem like hooey but take a moment to think about how it feels when your relationship is at its best. You smile at each other more. You may laugh more when together. At a party you may catch each other's eye and hold the stare for a moment, both knowing what that means. To be able to enjoy intimacy again definitely has an impact on many aspects of your everyday life. But how do you regain this intimacy when your body seems to be betraying you? How do you broach this subject with your doctor?

Women are very hesitant to speak to their doctors about intimate issues. One survey by Parish, Nappi, and Krychman showed that less than half of women suffering from vaginal atrophy or painful intercourse after menopause mentioned it at their visit. Regardless of their inability to discuss the problem with their physician, the survey showed thirty-four percent experienced a negative effect on self-esteem and forty-two percent influenced mood. They were clearly emotionally distressed by the condition of painful intercourse! Fifty five percent reported a negative effect on intimacy, and forty seven percent admitted having an overall negative effect on their relationship. Sixty two percent showed lower confidence. Clearly, the consequences of this issue are monumental in women's lives, yet more than half the time, it is not discussed. Therefore, it is still so underserved and under addressed. Women often say that when they did mention it to their doctor, they were appeased or dismissed. The reason is likely that the provider felt like they did not have any solution to offer.

Many women who experience urinary leakage think it is something they just have to live with, even though articles show that up to forty five percent of women will avoid intimacy due to fear of leaking. Once again, women fail to share this problem during their yearly visit and rarely will seek treatment for the issue in and of itself. Women need to feel free to bring up the problem and be offered a valid plan of action to improve the quality of life.

As you read further keep in mind four questions.

1. How could this help me?
2. If I fixed this problem, how would it affect my relationship?
3. If I got this treatment, how would it change my everyday life?
4. Why should I suffer with this condition for one more day if there are such easy and painless solutions?

PART 2

Chapter 4

'I't's All Wrong Down There

When did you first realize you were a girl? When did you notice how you were different than your brother or your father? It is at a very young age that gender identity starts, and this is not due to hormones, initially, but due to cultural norms. The mother usually begins identifying the infant as a baby boy or girl. The child then begins to relate to the cultural expectations. You were dressed accordingly. That was just the beginning. Have you ever wondered what happens as you develop and grow into women experiencing daily life changes?

Development

The first physiologic change women experience is menarche, or the initiation of menses. This is the beginning of the reproductive years and is hormonally driven. A fully mature woman meets the level of maturity called Tanner stage V. This is full sexual development with development of the breast tissue and female hair, along with ovarian function, including ovulation. Girls usually get their period for the first time between the ages of ten to sixteen, with thirteen being the average age. This makes a woman fertile, meaning she is now able to get pregnant and have a baby!

Pregnancy

With pregnancy, the physiologic changes are significant. The growth of the uterus over nine months accompanies weight gain due to the developing fetus and accumulation of amniotic fluid. Women have a fifty percent increase in blood volume in order to support the pregnancy. It is through the placenta that the baby receives all its nourishment. The human body undergoes changes such as relaxation of pelvic muscles and bony structures to allow the passage of the baby through the birth canal. The long-term changes following pregnancy can include direct damage to the tissue by episiotomy and/or tearing. The indirect laxity that occurs from stretching during vaginal birth results in decreased friction during intercourse and a feeling of looseness. So often, this is a complete surprise to a new mother. No one describes this during routine prenatal care. You go home with a weird jelly belly and a very sore bottom, and you begin to wonder if you will ever feel like your old self again.

Urinary Incontinence

If you ever noticed, the female openings

are really close together. With our structures so close, weakness in one area can cause problems right next door! The weakness of the tissue in the walls of the vagina causes relaxation of the urethra, which is the conduit of urine from the bladder. This can lead to all forms of urinary incontinence. One type is known as *urinary stress incontinence*. This is the leakage of urine associated with a cough, sneeze, or jump. Many women experience this during exercise or when jumping on a trampoline. This is extremely common, and yet women are ashamed to speak about it. The condition may limit a woman's activities and quality of life, yet she is reluctant to mention it to her doctor or even her friends. She thinks she is the only one with an extra pair of panties in her purse *just in case*!

Urge incontinence is when a woman may leak urine when she feels the *urge* to go void, before making it to the toilet. *Frequency* is simply an increase in the number of times she needs to void, causing inconvenience or even loss of sleep at night. Women have shared with me that they know where every bathroom is on their route to work or in every store at the mall. They admit to carrying a sweater not just for warmth but to cover their pants should an accident occur. Clinical studies have shown that forty-five percent of women who suffer from these conditions avoid sex. That is very damaging to a relationship.

You may have a combination of all these conditions known as *mixed urinary incontinence.* Due to these issues, there will be more adult diapers sold per year than baby diapers within the near future. These urinary symptoms progress and become more and more prevalent with age, after years of gravity pulling on the bladder and vaginal wall.

Female Sexual Dysfunction

A separate factor is female sexual dysfunction. This refers to the clinical conditions that relate to dysfunction of libido, arousal, or orgasm. They are defined in the professional reference book for psychiatric disorder classifications known as the DSM-5.

This includes:

Female orgasmic disorder - defined as a delay in, infrequency of, or absence of orgasm, or reduced intensity of orgasmic sensations during seventy-five to one hundred percent of sexual activity encounters. This ambiguous definition leaves it up to the patient and clinician to try to diagnose the condition.

Female sexual interest/arousal disorder - defined as absent or decreased sexual interest/arousal. This is determined by meeting three or more of the following criteria:

1. Decreased or absent interest in sexual activity

2. Decreased/absent sexual thoughts or fantasies

3. Reduced/no initiations of sexual activity or not responding to partner initiations.

4. Reduced/absent excitement or pleasure during seventy-five to one hundred percent of sexual activity events.

5. Reduced or absent interest/arousal in the context of any sexual cues

6. Reduced/absent genital or non-genital sensations during seventy-five to one hundred percent of sexual activity events.

To me, sexual interest and being able to be aroused are two very different conditions. I am not sure why these get lumped together in the psychiatric definitions above. While sexual interest has a psychological component, arousal is more of a physical sensation associated with the touch of erogenous zones, such as the lips, neck, breasts, and genitalia.

Genito-pelvic pain/penetration disorder is a constant or repeated difficulty with:

1. Vaginal penetration during intercourse

2. Vaginal or pelvic pain during penetration
3. Significant fear/anxiety about vaginal or pelvic pain
4. Tensing the pelvic floor muscles during penetration attempt

They further characterize each condition as being lifelong or acquired and may vary in severity from mild to severe. Sadly, so much of the disease of female sexual dysfunction is viewed and evaluated as psychological. I wish to explain how there are physical, psychological, and situational aspects to sexuality. The female orgasmic system involves physical aspects that require attention throughout life.

Hormonal Influences

As women age and produce less and less testosterone and estrogen, tissues of the female genitalia undergo drastic changes. Women lose up to one percent of testosterone yearly over the age of thirty. Estrogen levels wax and wane between

changes in the blood vessels in the vaginal wall.
With the thinning of the blood vessels, there is
less fluid exuding into the vagina during sex. The
result is that sex feels as if the round hairbrush
you use to blow dry your hair is grating on your
vagina! However, if adequate estrogen reaches
the vessels, they will rebuild their integrity and
natural lubrication will return (not to mention
the anti-aging effect estrogen has on the skin!).

All these changes and conditions affect a
woman's quality of life and her interactive skills
on personal and professional levels. These issues
are rarely discussed or recognized as treatable.
Coworkers might ask if you are feeling well or
they might just turn away and pretend not to
notice the profuse perspiration dripping off your
face. Most women think they must live with
these situations as normal consequences of life
and aging. That is the biggest myth of all!

Before I start discussing treatments, it is
imperative to understand that genitalia are

ally experiencing discomforts while exercising or from chafing in clothing. The World Health Organization claims that any surgery on genitals is mutilation. In 2007, the American college of Ob/Gyn (ACOG) made a statement that they did not recognize the procedures that minimize the size of labia because they were not supported by research evidence. Fortunately, more evidence-based reports are being published to prove the efficacy of some of these procedures.

The ACOG has released a new opinion easing their stance on the procedures as they become more and more popular and show benefits. There are four moral principles that separate rejuvenation procedures from mutilation. The first is non-maleficence, meaning "do no harm." Responsible providers do not do procedures that are not necessary. The second is autonomy, which means the patient must be at least eighteen years old and in sane mind to give informed consent and understand the risks and benefits. The third is that the doctor must never do the procedure for only monetary gain; there must be a medical indication. The last is that if the physician does not feel it is necessary despite the patient's desires, the procedure is not performed. The doctor must follow her gut in these situations. These principles make it evident this is not an immoral treatment.

The next important fact to observe is that there are no abnormal anatomic variations in female genitalia barring congenital anomalies; we are all "normal." There have been attempts to evaluate the average size of labia minora, as this is a common area where women seem to desire alteration. With studies, it was concluded the average is two centimeters with variation from one half to five centimeters.

A common complaint from women is that enlarged labia show in clothing and can protrude out of bathing suits, causing embarrassment. These inconvenient situations add public distress for many women. As a result, the reduction of the size of the labia minora is the most frequently sought-out treatment. If enlarged, labia might get in the way during exercise, like riding a bike or spinning, or can cause difficulty wearing certain types of clothing.

Another issue that causes embarrassment and daily frustration for women is urinary incontinence. Women who experience urinary accidents in public can feel socially ostracized. If there are simple, non-invasive, painless procedures to correct these issues, they are certainly not mutilation any more than the traditional procedures used to surgically repair a weak bladder. The standard of care in the past was the placement of meshes in the form of a sling beneath the bladder; in many cases, these eroded through the vaginal walls, resulting in more problems than the women had in the first place. This required the removal of some devices from the market and class action suits. The controversy around genital procedures stems from misunderstanding and simple ignorance. These valuable treatments are becoming popular in the growing field of cosmetic gynecology, also known as aesthetic gynecology, vaginal rejuvenation, or as I like to refer to it, *restorative gynecology*. They are not mutilation, but valid procedures that need to be added to the universal armamentarium.

Chapter 5

'N'ope! I Do Not Know What to Call That

To aid in understanding the description of the treatments, we will now explore the normal female anatomical structures. As I mentioned earlier, it is important to remember that variations in size, shape, and color are completely normal.

Here is a brief glossary of female anatomy:

Internal Organs

- Uterus: The uterus is a pear-shaped, female sex organ that has thick muscular walls. The uterus is where the fetus is housed until it is ready for birth. The lining of the uterus is the source of menstrual blood, and sheds if pregnancy does not occur. The bleeding is known as a monthly period.

- Ovary: The ovaries are the two main hormone-producing organs that hang out by the uterus. They release hormones like estrogen, progesterone, and testosterone, regulate the menstrual cycle, and support pregnancy.

- Fallopian tubes: Fallopian tubes are the roadway through which eggs pass from an ovary to the uterus. There is one ovary and one tube on each side of the uterus. The fallopian tubes have finger-like projections that receive chemical signals to identify the ovary and capture the egg that is released.

External Structures

- Vulva: The vulva is all the female stuff you see. Here you see the labia and the vagina (sometimes called the vestibule), the labia majora (outer lips), the labia minora (inner lips), and the clitoris. The opening of the vagina is surrounded by the hymen.

- Hymen: The hymen is the soft tissue ring that guards the vagina. When spoken of as "intact," this means it has not been torn in any way. Typically, an intact hymen implies virginity. The hymen has been known to tear with bike riding, horseback riding, and tampon use, as well as with sex. These tears in a hymen are varied and unique to each woman.

- Clitoris: The clitoris is the spot that gives sexual pleasure. There are eight-thousand nerve endings in the female clitoris, double that of the male penis. Its only purpose is for pleasure!

- Labia majora: The labia majora are the larger outer folds of the vulva. They may act as bumpers or padding for the genitalia. With aging, this area seems to lose fat and the skin may sag. It may look like a flat tire. This change may cause discomfort with sex or certain activities, like cycling.

- Labia minora: The labia minora are two small folds of soft tissue on each side of the opening into the vagina. These may vary in size, color, and shape. This is the anatomy that women seem to be most self-conscious about, causing them to seek cosmetic consultation and alteration. Their main function is to aid in the streaming of urine.

- Cervix: The cervix is the mouth of the womb. This is the area that is sampled during a pap smear. It is also responsible for cyclical vaginal discharge. The cervical mucus changes with the monthly physiological hormonal milieu.

- Vagina: The vagina is the tunnel that leads to the uterus or womb. The vagina is used for penetrating intercourse. It is lined by moist tissue known as mucosa, like the inside of the mouth. It has natural folds that can stretch and accommodate almost anything that enters it, whether that be a baby or a sexual partner. The walls have collagen, elastin, and blood vessels that each contribute to its optimal function.

- Urethra: This is the small tube that works as the exit for urination from the bladder. It sits just below the clitoris. Unfortunately, in women, the urethra is rather short. Therefore, it is so common to get urinary tract infections after sex; sex increases the opportunity for bacteria to travel up the urethra and into the bladder.

- Skene's Glands: These are small glands on either side of the urethra. It is believed to be where a woman ejaculates from. Some woman may release fluid with orgasm much like a man, colloquially known as squirting.

- G-Spot: This is an invisible area described as a cluster of soft tissue generally found on the front wall of the vagina. This is an area that is viewed as part of the female orgasmic system. Scientifically, this area has been elusive and controversial. The question is, "does it actually exist?" Women who have one certainly will insist that it is definitely there.

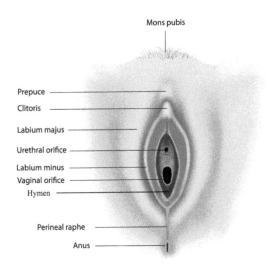

Chapter 6

'T'rim and Stitch All That

The Surgical Approach

t is time for some fun! You will now read stories typical of women you know or maybe even yourself. Surgical treatments will then be explained that are used to solve the predicament.

Labiaplasty

Case: Sally, a forty-seven-year-old woman who has just gone through a divorce, comes in with the complaint that she has always been self-conscious of the fact that one side of her labia minora is much larger than the other. She feels unattractive and ashamed of it. Everyone has been encouraging her to go on a dating site, but she hesitates. It has been years since she dated, and she would be so embarrassed to be seen naked. She wants to permanently correct the "weirdness" she has dealt with her whole life. She undergoes labiaplasty and is very pleased. When she shares with her eighteen-year-old daughter that she has had this done, her daughter confides that she too feels uncomfortable with the asymmetry of her labia minora. She calls for an appointment and has the same procedure.

Labiaplasty is the set of procedures done to decrease the size of the labia minora in order to solve the issues associated with discomfort and embarrassment. There are a few different ways this can be done, depending on the desired result. There is a trim technique that simply trims off the edge. Alternatively, the wedge technique preserves the natural edge of the labia while reducing overall size.

There are many possible complications with surgery. One must consider there is always the risk of needing additional surgery and a possibility of scarring and change in sensation. It is also important to consider that recovery from such a procedure includes six weeks of decreased activity, with the first two weeks being particularly critical in avoiding excessive walking. Intercourse is absolutely forbidden for these six weeks. It is similar to having a baby, but without the "taking care of the newborn" part. The results can be rather lovely, but the experience is intense.

Perineoplasty

Case: Justine, a thirty-five-year-old woman, comes to the office complaining that after giving birth vaginally, nothing has been the same. She feels like the opening to her vagina is large and gaping. During sex, she feels no sensation. She cannot feel anything in the G-spot anymore. She fears that her partner can feel the difference and may find her unattractive and stray. Upon examining her, the doctor notices that the episiotomy never healed correctly, and the area known as the introitus is indeed gaping. The procedure to correct this would be a perineoplasty.

Women often experience a feeling of looseness or laxity after childbirth. A woman will either rip or receive an episiotomy during vaginal childbirth, and once this occurs, she no longer feels the same. Episiotomy is the intentional cutting of the vaginal opening done by the doctor during delivery to help fit the baby out. It is accompanied by loss of sensation and sexual pleasure. The common thought is that since the lower one third of the vagina is where you have the most sensation, that is where the tightening should occur. The procedure is basically cutting a new episiotomy, re-approximating the muscles in the lower third of the vagina, and removing excess skin or previous scars. Once again, the recovery is six weeks of no intercourse and exercise. The complication here is possible pain in the area of tightened tissue or scarring. Sometimes it is difficult to judge how much tissue to remove and the doctor may over tighten, which can make having sex painful rather than pleasurable.

Cystocele and Rectocele Repair

Case: The receptionist says, "Ms. Jones just called because there is something hanging out of her vagina! What should I tell her?" Her doctor immediately responds, "Please have her come in to be seen." What is happening? The vagina is acting like a hernia! The uterus and the bladder and the rectum are all protruding from the vaginal opening. Due to gravity and damage to the tissues of the pelvic floor during childbirth, Ms. Jones has developed herniation of any or all of these organs: the bladder, the cervix, the uterus, and the rectum. This is known as prolapse, and surgery is one way to treat this. The extent of tissue damage is important for the doctor to evaluate to best decide the appropriate fix.

These are more traditional procedures that are used to reduce over stretched tissue that develops after childbirth due to laxity in the walls of the vagina. They involve making incisions in the front and back walls of the vagina. The recovery is six weeks of no intercourse and no heavy lifting. It is my opinion that if the vaginal tissue is maintained utilizing the new, less invasive techniques, these operations may never be necessary. I am also concerned that these procedures cut right through the g-spot, possibly destroying this tissue.

Mesh Procedures

Case: Mary arrives at the office and, just from the drive and the walk from the parking lot to the entrance, her pad is already wet; she feels as though she cannot hold her urine at all. When she is seen by her doctor, she's told she had a *dropped bladder*. She thinks, at fifty-five, this isn't a way to live. The pads she has to wear are expensive and by the end of the day, she feels like everyone can smell her. She feels like a baby with a wet diaper neglected by her mommy. When her partner wants to be romantic, she refuses his advances because she feels dirty and smelly. There is no time for spontaneity because she has to jump in the shower before she feels ready for intimacy. Sometimes he is asleep by then or the moment has just passed. She needs this fixed! The doctor explains that conservative measures like Kegel's will not be enough and surgery is necessary. In most extreme cases, there is still a need for corrective surgery.

The mesh procedures involve placing a sling under the bladder neck to act like a hammock. The attempt is to use the sling to return the anatomy to the proper spot and return the support and function. These procedures have been used for at least a decade, but have had serious complications, to the point that they have been removed from the market in the USA. New versions of this procedure may be offered by specialists and use either an autograft (tissue from the patient's tendons) or animal sources to create the supportive sling under the bladder.

If there is significant amount of damage to the vagina, it may be necessary to have invasive surgery. Not everyone can be treated with the minimally invasive procedures. The less invasive procedures will be explored in following chapters.

Clitoral Hood Reduction

Case: Joanie, a fifty-year-old woman makes an appointment with her doctor because she finally realizes that there is a way to improve her ability to orgasm. She has had a very difficult time climaxing all her sexual life but with recent hormonal changes, she is finding it almost impossible to climax. Upon exam, the clitoral hood is very thick, and it is hard to see the clitoris. Even if she is with the most skilled lover, and he knows to expose the most sensitive tip, it does not seem to be possible. The correction is ideally surgical in this case and includes removing the excess tissue making the glans or outer tip of the clitoris easily assessable.

This relatively quick in-office procedure can remove the skin over the clitoris. A small incision is made in the area where the extra tissue is covering the anatomy. It is excised and dissolving stitches are placed to close the incision. The down time is about two weeks. No exercise or intercourse is allowed for this period of time. Possible complication is either infection or disruption of the stitches, as in any surgery. The unique risk in this case is removal of too much skin and over stimulation may occur. In that

Chapter 7

'I'n the Simplest Ways

Regenerative Procedures

Fat Grafting of the Labia Majora

Case: Forty-eight-year-old Connie enters the doctor's office, ashamed of how her genitals have changed. "Look at what happens when I stand! The skin just hangs! It never looked like this before. Now, when I have sex it feels like he is hitting right into my bones. I have lost all my padding. Is there anything that can be done?"

This procedure requires a two-step process. The fat is harvested from one place in the body and transferred to the labia. The fat is grafted by using liposuction. The patient and the doctor will decide where they would like to have the fat harvested. In one common scenario, the fat comes from the enlarged mons pubis. The mons pubis is the fatty pad that lies over the pubic bone in the front of the body between the legs. If this is possible, then it addresses two issues at once. If excess fat is not found in the mons, then either the abdomen or outer thigh are chosen. The fat is then processed for return to the body. The fat is reintroduced into the labia majora, restoring the fullness. The recovery is rather simple, except that the areas of liposuction or where the fat was harvested must be kept under pressure for two weeks. This requires a garment like a body shaper to keep the area compressed and must be worn day and night. The result appears natural and long lasting.

Platelet Rich Plasma

Case: Emily, a forty-two-year-old, comes to share that she has *never* had an orgasm. She loves her husband but has never been bold enough to share with him that she has never reached orgasm when they are together. She shares that when she was in grade school, she experienced a fall on the monkey bars that ripped her apart. Since then, she has lacked sensation in the clitoral area. Upon exam there are absolutely no signs of scarring or anything abnormal. Following the O- Shot™, she experiences an orgasm for the first time. She shares that when an orgasm started to happen, she felt a sense of panic not knowing what was occurring. Now, the ability to be able to experience that natural pleasure with the man she loves has reignited her passion. She expresses that she feels like she was deaf and can hear music for the first time.

Thanks to the absolute genius of Dr. Charles Runels, the use of platelet rich plasma in genitalia has been discovered. The multiple uses of this elixir of life are changing people's lives worldwide. Platelet Rich Plasma (PRP) has been used for many years in several areas of medicine. It harnesses the healing qualities of the portion of our blood carrying the platelets, and its applications are endless. When doctors were exploring how the body naturally heals, they focused on the clear, yellow tinged fluid that extrudes from a wound. They discovered that platelets, when exposed to injury, excrete alpha granules. These granules contain growth factors that induce the body to build new tissue to repair the damage. PRP also can activate natural stem cells to regenerate the tissue needed in the area of the injury.

Scientists then discovered how to isolate, concentrate, and return PRP to the site of injury. With FDA-approved kits and FDA-approved centrifuge machines, this is simply accomplished by drawing blood from the patient's arm. The blood is then processed in the centrifuge (a machine that spins the blood and allows the different components to separate) and returned to the area in need of treatment. Due to weight differences, the red blood cells will sink to the bottom, and the magic platelets rise to the top, separating like oil and vinegar. The results have been barely short of miraculous! The *O-Shot*™ is the trademarked procedure used to improve the sensation of the female genitalia and to help build new tissue around the urethra. The results of this painless procedure are greatly improved orgasmic function and urinary continence. I refer you to http://www.elitedaily.com/women/the-o-shot-for-better-orgasms/1489532 written by one of my patients.

PRP may also be used to fill the labia majora instead of the fat transfer. Per Dr. Runels, the *Vampire Winglift*™ is the trademarked procedure which combines hyaluronic acid and PRP to fill the labia to return them to a normal plumpness. This acts as a bumper during intercourse protecting the pubic symphysis. When labia are plump and full, it prevents them from folding into the vagina and getting in the way during intercourse.

Dermal fillers for labial plumping

Dermal fillers that contain hyaluronic acid have been used extensively for aesthetics of the face. They are used to improve the appearance of facial wrinkles and sagging skin. With hyaluronic acid's filling capability already established, it was logical to attempt filling the labia majora with these products. This works nicely, however some patients will experience temporary lumps or nodules. The results will last as long as it takes the individual to metabolize the product, usually is around nine to twelve months.

Supportive Therapies

Carboxy Therapy

This procedure aids in replenishing tissue with carbon dioxide (CO_2). The ultimate effect is improved oxygenation that enriches the quality of the tissue. Carboxy is used to improve vaginal blood flow, hence improving lubrication. It may also aid in wound healing and may be injected directly into a surgical scar, such as a cesarean section wound.

LED Light Therapy

The LED therapy is an at-home treatment or office treatment. It is used intra-vaginally and emits LED light helping to improve vaginal pH or acid/base balance. There are LED devices that are used externally to stimulate collagen development and aid in skin tightening of the external surface of the vulva. It may also work to improve wound healing following any surgery. It has been used in other specialties for acne treatment and other dermatological conditions.

Hormone Therapy

As a woman ages, the main cause of vaginal issues is the lack of estrogen and testosterone. There are a lot of issues to consider when thinking about using therapy to replace these hormones. In 2002, a study known as The Woman's Health Initiative showed that oral synthetic estrogen and synthetic progesterone increases the risk of cardiovascular disease, stroke, breast cancer, and dementia. This caused worldwide panic, and women stopped using hormones. The consequence has been a huge detriment to women. Thankfully, since that original study, it has been discovered that the transdermal use of hormones, especially bioidentical hormones, does not have the same risk. Ongoing studies, such as the KEEPS study or Biol Sex Differ.

Andrea Iorga, Christine M. Cunningham, Shayan Moazeni, Gregoire Ruffenach, Soban Umar, and Mansoureh Eghbali are showing the benefits of estrogen in women when used appropriately. Bioidentical hormones are plant derived products that are chemically identical to what the human body produces. There are pharmaceutical-grade estrogen and progesterone hormones available, but there are no commercial testosterone products available for women in the USA. For men, large pharmaceutical companies produce testosterone in gels, creams, injections, and pellets. The only way to replace testosterone in women is from specialty pharmacies; these pharmacies will create similar preparations for women to the doctor's specific recommendations. The compounded hormones are tailored to the individual by using blood levels. The levels are followed, and dosages are modified if needed.

The benefit of hormone therapy is to improve overall quality of life. Using estrogen will decrease mood swings, hot flashes, night sweats, dry skin, and vaginal dryness. Using testosterone improves energy levels, mental alertness, the ability to build muscle, quality of sleep, and sexual sensations, while it also decreases body fat. A philosophy to follow here is to optimize our aging health. Life expectancy with medical advances is extending and living better for longer is the goal. The life expectancy of a baby born in 2020 is one hundred and twenty years old. According to the article written by Dr. Kaare Christensen in the *Lancet*, it is time to begin to live better.

Intravaginal Hormones

Some patients do not require systemic hormones or just prefer not to use them. In this case, there are many preparations for intravaginal use. One is a silicone ring that delivers local estrogen to the tissues over three months and then is removed, discarded, and replaced with a new one. Estrogen can also be delivered as vaginal cream preparations, tablets, or gel caps. There are also vaginal suppositories of DHEA, which is a hormone released by the adrenal gland. When used intravaginally daily, the cells break DHEA down into estrogen and testosterone. This works as an indirect way to replace the local estrogen. All these therapies help, but doses are kept very low to avoid systemic absorption. Maintaining this balance to avoid systemic estrogen levels limits the dosing and may not totally repair the tissue to the level needed to make intercourse comfortable. The effects are therefore somewhat limited by the need to avoid the hormones being absorbed into the blood stream. This results in sub-optimal rejuvenation of the vaginal walls, decreasing the effectiveness.

Skin Lightening

Yes! Many women become self-conscious of the color of the skin on their vulva. Due to friction, the area darkens over time. With the popularity of waxing and laser hair reduction to achieve complete hair removal, the skin changes are more evident. It is thought that, due to easy accessibility to online porn, women are getting ideas of what they think is the cultural norm for what their vaginas should look like. Women seek out ways to change the color of the skin on the labia and in the creases by their thighs and around the anus. There are many topical agents, lotions, and potions to be used for skin lightening. Many doctors have come up with personal brands and protocols for the skin treatments in this zone. Chemical peels are also used for changing the color of the skin. All the treatments are aimed at decreasing the activity of melanosomes, which are the cells in the skin that get activated either by light or friction to produce melanin, causing skin to darken just like tanning. The topical therapies work well and may be augmented with laser therapy, which will be explained in the next chapter on energy-based devices.

Chapter 8

'M'aybe Energy Has Promise

Lasers

C ase: Cloe, at fifty-three-years-old, has entered menopause and is having terrible pain with intercourse. She does not want to tell her husband because she fears he will think it is his fault. With each week that goes by, it is getting worse and worse. She fears that soon she will not be able to hide her discomfort. It feels like razor blades every time he moves inside her when they are being intimate. Can he see the horror in her face? No more candlelight for them, she thinks. The darker the better so she can hide her pain. The problem is that she is noticing her whole body tighten in fear of his touch. He must be able to sense that. Her reaction is involuntary, but automatic now. What are her options?

One of the greatest discoveries was that lasers such as fractionated ablative CO_2 lasers can be modified to be used to treat the vagina and vulva. These painless procedures are fast and extremely effective to return a very natural sense of lubrication, alleviating vaginal dryness. The laser makes micro-injuries along the anterior vaginal wall, causing new collagen and blood vessels to be created that support the bladder neck. Patients report improvement in urinary incontinence. When the laser's modified hand piece is used externally, it results in skin tightening of the labia majora. Using the light scan attachment, skin lightening may be accomplished with a series of treatments. The down time required following these procedures is a total of three days of no sex. No other restrictions are necessary. The treatments are done one month apart for three months and once yearly for maintenance. The result is leak free, well lubricated, and comfortable sex. Turn the lights on or light those candles!

Using the erbium laser in the vagina has been shown to have similar effects. The difference is that the erbium does require some numbing cream to be used during the procedure. This simply makes the procedure take a little longer to allow the numbing cream to take effect. The down time is like that of the CO_2 laser. The treatment requires three visits one month apart and one treatment for yearly maintenance.

Thulium Laser

A newer usage of thulium laser may be used to aid in skin lightening. The treatment is painless and requires three visits spaced two to four weeks apart. Results are very satisfying. It is so simple that there is not much more that needs to be said. It will be rather popular once doctors realize the benefits and women start requesting it.

Radio frequency for treating the vagina and the external genitalia

The original radio frequency device popularized by Dr. Red Alinsod has been available for the past few years. It is a monopolar device used to create a tightening sensation. The downside is that it takes up to twenty-five to forty-five minutes to perform, with the probe going in and out of the vagina. It is less expensive than laser treatments, so it may be a valid alternative when cost is a limiting factor.

Since the advent of the original monopolar device, there is an explosion on the market of all variations, including some that use bipolar radio frequency. Some combine cooling or cryotechnology together with heating radio frequency. These are all new to the market and remain to be evaluated for efficacy or how well they work on the vaginal tissue. The treatments are done once a week or every other week for three to four visits, and once a year for maintenance. The immediate result is a sense of tightening and increased blood flow. These effects are initially short-lived; however, the full result will occur within six months. New collagen, elastin, and blood vessels are created.

High Intensity Focused Electromagnetic Technology (HIFEM)

This discovery of how to strengthen muscle in such a simple way has revolutionized the treatment of urinary incontinence and sexual satisfaction. FDA-approved for the treatment of urinary incontinence, devices that use HIFEM allow women to sit on a chair fully clothed and retrain their pelvic muscles.

The pelvic muscles form the floor of our torso; they could be referred to as the cradle of civilization. These muscles are weakened by pregnancy, aging, and childbirth. Strengthening the muscles gives back control; control of urine as well as the ability to engage these muscles during intimacy. This can enhance enjoyment for both you and your partner. The machine works by using electromagnetic energy emitted from a tesla magnet in the chair. The energy causes 11,200 super maximal contractions of all the pelvic floor muscles. It is like doing thousands of perfect Kegel exercises. Kegels have been recommended for forty years by every gynecologist. The problem with the exercise is that most women never do them correctly or frequently enough, leading to frustration for most people who have attempted this approach. The HIFEM treatment requires two visits a week for three weeks. The newly developed muscle will last for at least six months, but maintenance is recommended every four to six months with a treatment or two.

When and where necessary, any and all these procedures can be combined to address every issue.

Chapter 9
'A'bout the Future

Where we go from here is extremely exciting. New restorative therapies using stem cells derived from our own fat or bone marrow are revolutionizing medicine as we know it. Extensive research is being done, and the applications of this methodology are endless. You heard it here first. Follow the progress of international organizations listed below:

- The American Aesthetic Association, www.ameriaa.com

- The International Society of Regenerative Medicine, www.isregen.org
- The Cellular Medicine Association, www.oshot.com
- The CIMEG, www.cimegmadrid.com
- The International Society of Cosmetic Gynecology, Aesthetics, and Research, www.iscgyn.com
- The European Society of Aesthetic Gynecology, www.esag.org
- Organicell, www.organicell.com
- StemGenn, www.stemgenn.com

The amazing contributions by these genius doctors around the world are unimaginable.

The field is expanding, and knowledge is empowering. Below are some areas to keep an eye on.

Stem Cell Therapy

Stem cells can be used to treat a disease or condition. The best known is bone marrow transplant, which has been used for cancer treatment for decades. The more recent uses are controversial and were banned in the USA in the past for ethical reasons, mostly because at one point, stem cells were being derived from embryos. Today, stem cells can be gathered from a patient's own bone marrow or fat, amniotic membranes, or cord blood. Stem cells are being used internationally to treat ovarian failure and lack of sperm, reversing infertility in men and women. They are also improving treatments for neurodegenerative conditions, heart disease, and diabetes. The uses are endless.

Exosomes

Exosomes are the latest advancement in regenerative medicine. Exosomes are growth factors and anti-inflammatory chemicals released by stem cells. They may be even more important than stem cells because they help cells communicate via messenger RNA (mRNA), which stimulates new protein growth. Exosomes can be derived from fluid in amniotic tissues. This means that the patient does not have to have a procedure to collect exosomes; they are being collected from the discardable tissues that surround a baby during pregnancy that are universally compatible with all people after the baby is born. These tissues are an infinite source of the exosomes.

ExtraCellular Matrix

This is the collection of molecules released by cells that provides structural and biochemical support to the cells that it surrounds. The use of Matrix remains to be seen but holds promise in magnifying the effects of the aforementioned therapies.

Vitamin Infusions

Intravenous therapy is available at integrative or functional medicine practices that give specific vitamin treatments directly into your bloodstream. This is an anti-aging and energy boosting therapy. It is a way to get super charged by vital vitamins like Vitamin D or B complex.

Peptides

Several peptide treatments have become popular in anti-aging medicine. The International Peptide Society is a great resource for details about the multiple uses of peptides in reparative medical therapy. Peptides are small chains of amino acids shorter than would be considered a protein and can have anti-aging effects by improving our immune system. There are peptides that influence natural growth hormone, the immune system, or tissue repair. They can be used to enhance tendon or muscle healing. The full scope of peptide therapy is yet to be realized.

The field of knowledge surrounding the idea of optimizing aging health has been expanding.

On the technological side of development, engineers are at work discovering ways to use lasers, HIFEM, Radio Frequency, and combined technologies in a single device to improve safety and efficacy. With the awareness of what is at hand now and what is to come, you can make a more informed plan of treatment to address your complaints. The field is expanding so rapidly that some devices are already obsolete within months of hitting the market, much like cell phones. You buy the newest, greatest phone and one month later, an even better phone is released. That is the speed of change in the field of female sexual health. Sit back, relax, keep your seat belt on, and enjoy the ride… just do not stay on the sidewalk!

NEW TOPICAL PRODUCTS

There are a few amazing products that are soon to hit the market. They have been shown to increase blood flow to female genitalia. They may be the first clinically proven topical agents to improve the quality of female sexual response. It cannot get easier than that! Apply twenty minutes before sex and enjoy.

Chapter 10

'C'ombinations to Conjure

C ase: Theresa, a fifty-nine-year-old who has had four vaginal births, comes in with urinary stress incontinence, urge incontinence, and frequency. She needs to make sure she knows where the restrooms are wherever she goes and frequently empties her bladder to try to avoid accidents. She wears dark colors in case of a problem and uses pads when in public in case of leakage. She adds that she is having vaginal laxity with decreased satisfaction during intercourse and a fear that she may leak.

She avoids sex with her partner because of fear of embarrassment.

Solution:

- Vaginal Laser
- Radio Frequency Intravaginal
- HIFEM
- O-Shot™

This is a typical patient, and not a unique circumstance. Many women face these issues every day! To renew her confidence and restore her sexual enjoyment, we will combine many of the different procedures I have described in previous chapters. A woman like this would benefit from a vaginal laser treatment to improve vaginal tone and increase blood vessels around the bladder neck. This will help to reinforce the sphincter of the bladder to hold urine. She will also benefit from radio frequency of the vagina to have an immediate sense of tightness, as well as improved collagen, elastin, and blood vessels six months down the road. The HIFEM technology will strengthen the Kegel muscles, giving her better voluntary control of urine and tightness. Finally, the O-Shot™ or PRP will help tissues grow at the bladder neck, enhancing the other energy-based device treatments – like added fertilizer. So, when the patient's situation is complicated with several issues, the additive effect of various therapies may be needed to correct the situation.

Case: Jen, a fifty-two-year-old, presents two years into menopause with vaginal dryness and painful intercourse exacerbated with loss of sensation and inability to reach orgasm. She has had to avoid sex due to the discomfort, and it is putting a wedge between her and her partner.

Solution:

• Vaginal Laser
• O-Shot™
• Hormone Optimization

In this situation, the immediate fix is the vaginal laser followed by the V-Shot, all possible at the same visit. If she has had a recent normal pap smear, laser treatments may be started. The next step is to have her hormones evaluated for testosterone. If her levels are particularly low, then she may be a candidate for pellet therapy. This treatment will be tailored to her specific needs. The difference in this circumstance is her specific lack of desire or libido. Desire can be partially a psychological issue. Testosterone works on desire areas of the brain and will increase libido. Optimizing her hormonal status, boosted by the miracles of PRP delivered by the O-Shot™ and by improvement in blood flow to the vaginal walls via laser therapy, will restore her satisfying sexual function.

Case: Laurie is forty-five-years-old and has no libido, lack of sensation, and vaginal laxity following three vaginal births. She describes extreme fatigue and weight gain. Feeling miserable, she is withdrawing from everyone important in her life. She feels a profound melancholy, like a black cloud following her around. She lacks energy to go to the gym, and the weight gain is adding to the vicious cycle.

Solution:

- Thyroid Hormone
- Testosterone optimization
- Radio Frequency internally and externally
- HIFEM

First, she needs a hormone evaluation. With her testosterone level undetectable and signs of hypothyroidism, her hormones must be optimized. In the meantime, she will benefit from intravaginal and vulvar radio frequency (RF). The last treatment for Laurie is the HIFEM Kegel chair treatment. The RF will increase her vaginal tone as well as tighten the skin on the exterior vulva. The hormones will improve libido, energy, and mood. The HIFEM will give the pelvic muscles strength to engage voluntarily during sex, lending a sense of tightness and increased blood flow to the area.

The cases go on and on, but the take-away message is that each woman is an individual and may require one or all the treatments available in order to address the issues she is experiencing. Another quandary is that over time, one problem may be corrected but a new issue may develop due to aging. Continuous maintenance of our sexual health is needed to keep active in the best working shape. It is a lot like getting a haircut or coloring our hair; it is not a one-and-done type of therapy. You need to keep up the visits, so your hair does not look disheveled. Just like your hairstyle might change over time, so do the personal needs of female sexuality.

Chapter 11

'Y'ou Are Ready for Action

You now know the natural, yet life altering changes women experience throughout their lives. Being informed of your own anatomy can help you understand where you need to be treated. With this simple knowledge, you can speak to your provider and explain the symptoms you are having.

You now have a knowledgeable foundation on the possible procedures that exist to address these issues. You know what to ask for depending on the condition you would like resolved, and you can customize your treatment to your own needs. It is my desire to educate women of the world so that they no longer have to suffer in silence. There are many options available to cure whatever ails you, and they are readily available and spreading fast around the world. Below, I include websites to aid in your exploration of providers well-versed in these therapies.

Visit:

- www.oshot.com
- www.iscgyn.com
- www.ameriaa.com
- www.organicell.com

You will want to find a doctor who is certified and credentialed in the treatments. In the USA, if your doctor has a valid license and insurance coverage, they can be trained to perform noninvasive procedures. Next, you may want to see how much experience the provider has had. The best scenario is if you already have a rapport with the doctor. Since sexual health is such a delicate and private subject, feeling comfortable and secure is of the utmost importance. If, for any reason, you do not feel relaxed in the clinical setting, it may be worth seeking a second opinion. In regard to any aspect of health, you should have confidence in your provider.

If you know the type of treatment you need, that may also guide your choice of provider. Not all doctors offer all therapies. Seeking a caretaker who can offer the specific device you want is key. Before choosing an office, make sure they have what you desire.

Cost may play a role as well. The most discouraging aspect of these procedures is that they are not covered by insurance. They are deemed experimental and cosmetic, so the insurance companies do not recognize them. In cities, the cost may be higher because rent and cost of doing business inflate the price. The experience and expertise of the provider may also influence the cost. You may have to weigh the situation and decide which features are most important to consider before making your appointment. The fee for consultation may be a consideration as well. Some offices will charge these fees, and some will not. Location and office hours will also be important, as repeat visits are required for some devices. Taking time off from work to make the appointment may have to figure into the equation.

Find a practice that feels right for you. This is your intimate health and all these parameters will need to balance out for you to have the greatest experience possible.

PART 3

Chapter 12

Agony to Ecstasy

Why did you never know that these treatments were even available?

To summarize what has been discussed in the previous pages:

1. Doctors shy away from the field due to misconception of mutilation
2. Patients do not discuss the problems with their doctor
3. Women are unaware that others are experiencing the same issues and suffer in silence

4. The technologies are deemed "aesthetic" instead of medical, and therefore are not mainstream and not readily available

5. Very few doctors are well versed in the field

6. My book was not written yet. (Just kidding!)

Medicine today is founded on evidence. That means that there are clinical trials proving the safety and efficacy of almost every treatment. Each country has its own version of a controlling body, such as the FDA in the USA that governs the use of devices. That being said, there are not a lot of prospective double-blind placebo studies completed on these treatments. The issue is that the devices being used are lasers and are energy-based, which makes offering a placebo treatment difficult; in other words, they are difficult to "fake." Additionally, the FDA has put restrictions on the manufacturer's ability to advertise due to the lack of evidence from large-scale, double-blind placebo studies. This limits the awareness of both the public and physicians, preventing women from accessing treatments that could change their lives for the better.

Studies supporting PRP are lacking due to difficulty in getting financial backing to fuel this research. PRP is a blood product, and therefore no large pharmaceutical company is producing it or funding research on it; your own body makes it! An added challenge is that any study on sexual satisfaction has a large placebo effect component, and this weakens the validity of the outcome or endpoints. The governing bodies in aesthetic and gynecological specialties are therefore hesitant to acknowledge the field. The trickle-down effect is that not many doctors are willing to jump in and forge the path. The crime here is that the women of the world are clamoring for help.

The devices used in the growing field of cosmetic gynecology are alterations of technologies that have been used for years in the field of aesthetic medicine. This makes the procedures fall into a category that is misgiving and misleading to both the doctor and the patient. Terms like "cosmetic" and "aesthetic" imply that these treatments are used merely for the appearance of the genitalia, when this couldn't be farther from the truth. The appearance is the least important aspect of this specialty; the crux of these treatments is their ability to improve function. Women deserve to have this function restored so that they no longer need to stress about urine leakage, and so that they can enjoy intimacy with their partners again. Although there are times when appearance does affect function, the final indication is always function. The problem is that many doctors and patients are confused by the "aesthetic" terminology and steer away from learning about the therapies.

Due to the ignorance about the purpose of the devices and treatments, there are very few doctors who have sought out training. There are several courses offered worldwide by those who have pioneered the procedures, and it is advised that doctors be properly certified and that patients identify their physician as being so educated.

I hope that this book will be a source for patients to be enlightened on a subject that was previously taboo, and I hope it will encourage more women and doctors alike to explore how to benefit from their newfound knowledge. I encourage you to share this knowledge with friends, family, and physicians. The more we talk about these topics, the more women will realize that they are not alone, and that they no longer need to suffer.

Conclusion

When you address the issues that have been holding you back from living the most fulfilled life you desire, you will be reborn. The metamorphosis will take place seamlessly and your wings will spread so you can soar. The inability to be intimate with your partner puts a serious damper on your happiness. If you are one of the fifty percent of women who have lack of confidence due to an inability to be or feel sexual, once this is returned, new emotions will bubble up.

You will remember the peaceful feeling in your soul that you can only experience when you know your relationship is solid and secure. Instead of occupying your time worrying about how to manage the pain or embarrassment of incontinence, you enjoy the simple pleasures of life. After pursuing the appropriate treatment, sex is comfortable, enjoyable, and desirable. You have never been closer to your partner and all your deepest fantasies are being realized every day. Your children feel the harmony in the household and seem to laugh more. The stresses from schoolwork are more manageable and less overwhelming for them. The positive energy between you as parents has an impact on the confidence and security of the children.

Feeling content at home allows you to flourish at work. You have more courage to face challenges and demands that seemed insurmountable when you were feeling inadequate.

With this newfound backbone, no goal is too difficult to achieve.

There is no reason to wait another moment to claim your life back. Stop suffering in silence and get the help you need.

Acknowledgments

I have so many people to be grateful for. I will begin with my mentors. The greatest mentors of all will be my family; my parents, my siblings, my aunts and uncles, and my cousins. I come from one of the most amazing families in the world. My siblings are all brilliant and successful, as are my cousins. We come from a long line of overachievers and philanthropists. My parents inspired me while they were alive, but I have felt their wind beneath my wings since they have passed on more strongly than ever.

Secondly, I must acknowledge that there is not one good doctor who does not have amazing nurses working beside them. I would be nothing without the talented and unbelievably caring nurses who have worked with me over the past 30 years. So, to Rena, Joyce, Cathy, Luanne, and Tina, I want to send out a heartfelt thank you for your unconditional support for me and all the patients that we cared for over the years. I could never forget the loyalty and contributions of the backbone of my practice: my supporting staff. Special acknowledgment must go to Isabel, Janet, Lexi, and Ally. None of my practices would be possible without your commitment and unlimited dedication and duty to our mission as a team to improve the lives of women.

I would be remiss not to acknowledge my dear friends. Without their strength and support and undying devotion, I could not be half the woman I am. You have kept me grounded and your honesty is your greatest attribute. I am blessed to have each and every one of you in my life. So, to Lorraine, Janet, Susanne, Germaine, Beth, Melanie, Lana, and Allison, I want to say you are a greater part of this book than you could ever imagine.

To my non-family mentors Dr. Charles Runnels, Darren Hardy, Dr. Ayman El Attar, Angela Lauria and the Author Incubator team, I want to say thank you for the faith you have placed in me. The knowledge and the genius that you have all shared has inspired me to achieve what I never would have imagined possible. You all continue to keep me moving forward each and every day.

Lastly to all the men who have touched my "life," I want to say thank you for showing me the importance of an intimate connection as a key factor in any human relationship. May you always feel the passion that fulfills your souls in all aspects of your life.

Thank you to David Hancock and the Morgan James Publishing team for helping me bring this book to print.

Sincerely,
Carolyn

Thank You Page

Wow! You made it to the end of Ultimate Intimacy! Thank you for completing the first step to a better life, both sexually as well as spiritually. To continue this path, I am offering an eight-week program. Please email your contact information to vivagyn@yahoo.com and I will personally share the details. I look forward to meeting you.

To get more information and for viewing pleasure, please subscribe to my YouTube channel Carolyn DeLucia, MD and follow me on

Instagram at dr.carolyndelucia. An even better choice is come on in to the VSPOT MediSpa nearest you! Visit www.vspotmedispa.com or www.vivarejuvenationcenter.com to schedule an appointment.

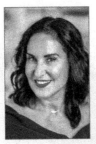

About the Author

D r. Carolyn DeLucia has been a board-certified OB/GYN in practice since 1992. She did her undergraduate studies at Rutgers College in New Jersey where she graduated with honors and Phi Beta Kappa. She went on to medical school at New York Medical College, followed by her internship and residency at Long Island Jewish Medical Center in New York. After several years of Obstetrics and Gynecology, she has evolved her practice to encompass gynecology and anti-aging medicine.

With her interest growing in preventative techniques, she opened ViVa Rejuvenation center in Hillsborough, New Jersey and is Medical Director of VSPOT Medispa in NYC. She focuses on signs of aging and performs non-invasive procedures to soften the evidence of time. Dr. DeLucia has expanded her attention to female sexual health and vaginal regenerative medicine, and this has become her mission. She welcomes patients to her practices with the hopes of making their lives better by ensuring optimized health and quality of longer life. She enjoys developing a caring and sincere relationship with all of her patients.

She is a faculty member for the Cellular Medicine Association and for the American Aesthetic Association and the International Society of Regenerative Medicine, and the Intimate Wellness Institute. She has lectured in Madrid, Montecarlo, India, Dubai, Qatar, Palo Alto, New York, Los Angeles, Las Vegas, Houston, San Francisco, Dallas, Orlando, Scottsdale, Boston, Fort Lauderdale, Atlanta, and Chicago for these associations.

www.vivarejuvenation.com

Email: vivagyn@yahoo.com

OFFICE:

ViVa Rejuvenation Center: +1 908 431 5849

Printed in the USA
CPSIA information can be obtained
at www.ICGtesting.com
JSHW011908040324
58553JS00005B/18

9 781642 799217